How To Lose Weight While Eating

Take Out -Take Away

My Fast Food Diet

PETER J MACDONALD

PETER MACDONALD

HOW DO YOU SUCCEED IN LIFE?

"MAKE GOOD DECISIONS"
HOW DO YOU MAKE GOOD DECISIONS?
"EXPERIENCE"
HOW DO YOU GAIN EXPERIENCE?
"MAKE BAD DECISIONS"

OR

YOU CAN LEARN FROM THE EXPERIENCE OF
OTHERS
WHO HAVE MADE THE GOOD AND BAD
DECISIONS
AND HAVE A TRACK RECORD YOU CAN LEARN
FROM.

Contents

About the Author

Fast food and food on the run has been the life of Peter MacDonald, whose business kept him out on the road on a daily basis for years. But when his weight took off in his middle age, it seemed like it would never stop it going up. Peter then began a journey that has seen him make lots of good decisions and lots of bad decisions, and gain a lot of experience in managing this monster that seemed to want to take over his life. Getting Fat.

In many ways Peter MacDonald is just your average working man, with an entrepreneurial twist. Married to his wife of 30 years, Sandra, with three adult children, Peter is the founder of the VeryDirtyCarpets Brand of cleaning products in the USA, and a successful business in Canberra, Australia, with VeryDirtyCarpet.com. He is also author of the children's joke book series "Best Joke Books for Kids", so it's a busy life.

Peter has taken the time to share his story in the hope that it might inspire people to make the journey to better health.

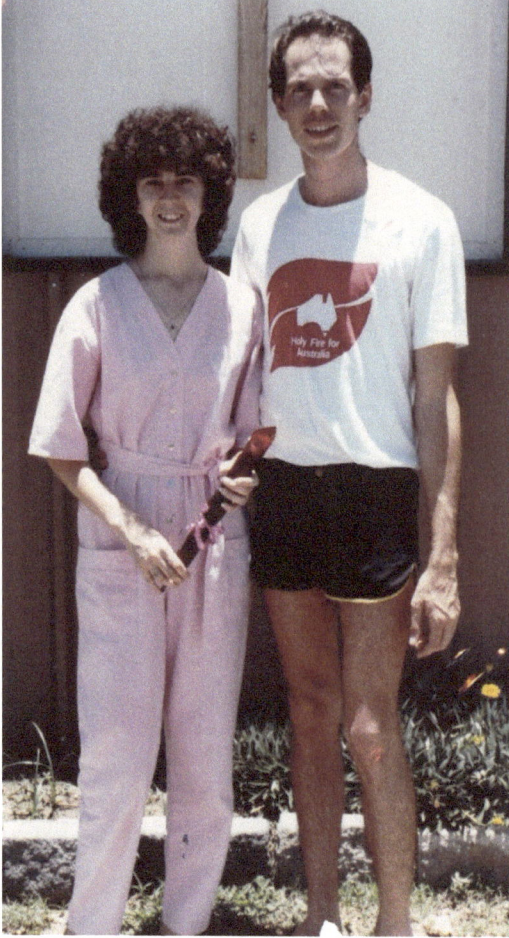

INTRODUCTION

You would say that much of my life is just normal. And in the same way that I am normal, I have struggled with the bogey man of mid-life weight gain. Since the age of 35, the normally skinny me, who at my wedding in 1986 weighed 143lbs/65 kg, began to put on weight slowly but steadily.

By the time I was 41, at my 15th wedding anniversary, my weight had crept up to 213lbs/97kg, 70lbs/32kg more than when I was married. When I was in my youth I could eat anything I liked, and not put on weight, but something had made my metabolism to slow down. It seemed like it didn't matter what I did now I would put on weight and inches around the middle.

It was around this time my wife, Sandra and I came across the book, "The Diet Revolution" by Dr. Atkins. I immediately warmed to the ideas in the Dr. Atkins book, and putting into practice his recommendations, I lost 44lbs/20kg in just over three months. But being human, high on the success of achieving this milestone, I started to celebrate, and over the next few months I put on much of the weight I had lost. Then sitting at about 204lbs/93kg, I was faced with a demoralizing decision. I had to look at doing it all over again.

Over the next 15 years I went through three or four cycles of losing weight and then putting it back on. The experience I gained during this time has allowed me to gain some insight into my own body, and while not an expert in the Weight Loss industry, I have become an expert on my own body, having come to know it intimately through these years.

You have to get to know your own body. No-one else knows your body like you do.

One of the challenges of dieting, as well as choosing the right food, is being in the right state of mind to be able to achieve success, and to continue to manage your diet once you have achieved your weight goal.

We have this incredible power to choose, to choose to accept fatalistically that this is just how it is, or to take control of our body, to choose what to eat and not to eat. The real battle goes on in our mind every day struggling with making these decisions.

I found that by using some common sense tools and wise implementation I was able to tackle the habits and patterns of thinking that had taken me prisoner.

My mother always told me when it came to

dating, "Fast to start, Fast to finish, Slow to start Slow to finish". This philosophy can be applied to dieting. Anything that is going to change us and get long term benefits is going to be slow to start and take consistent application. Any diet that promises fast results will by this definition give fleeting results. So this book is about gaining long term control of our diet and changing for the better our life style in general.

As we speak I have my weight down to below 84kg, and I have learnt to manage it at that weight and I am expecting to lose more on the coming months.

My other inspiration was Dr Michael Mosley, a medical journalist who has taken the time to shine the light on current research in the areas of fasting and calorie restriction, dieting and the medical implications of getting this area of your life in order.

My hope in sharing my story with you is that it might encourage you to take up the challenge. Gain better health, not pounds, by reducing the risk factors for losing weight and have it under control.

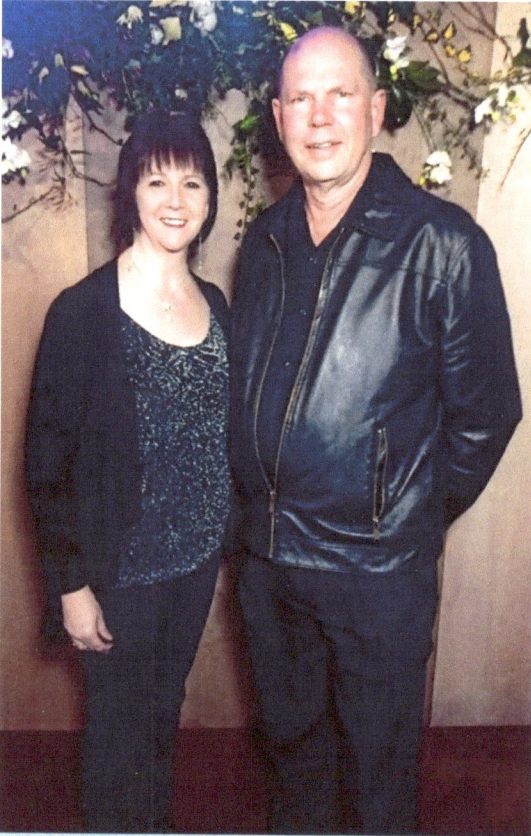

Peter and Sandra 2016
Peter at 190lbs/90 Kgs
Down from 213lbs/97Kgs
Ready to lode more.

Precaution

Some people may have medical conditions for which it is not wise to pursue weight loss without consulting a doctor. Please consult your doctor if you have any condition that may concern you.

The following book is based on what has worked for me, and on the recommendations of others with much more experience than I have.

Preface

You're not really listening if you haven't become aware of the tragedy that is enveloping western society and the battle with increasing waistlines, bellies, thighs and butts. And because of this many people and companies are trying to cash in on the perceived market for weight loss products, diets, fads and gizmo's to sell to desperate people who don't know where to turn to beat this menace.

I don't want to be just another voice in the blur of media, in the modern age, but what I do want to do is share what has helped me keep myself true and the battles I have had, but also share the success I have achieved.

Even if this book helps just one person get on top of the runaway weight gain they are struggling with then I will consider the effort of writing this book worthwhile.

In this book I want to:

1. Take a look at the problem that is confronting us.

2. Take a good look at the one who has the power to change it.

3. Take a look at what I have done to change my future.

4. Look at practical steps to take to effect change in our lives.

5. Identify a way to measure our success and monitor it on a daily basis.

6. Plan for the future once I have reached my weight goals so it doesn't happen again.

This book is not a novel, it is concise and hopefully clear to the reader so that, if they want to, they can make their own plans to succeed in their own battle of the bulge.

1 The Problem

At the risk of being painfully obvious, once most people reach a certain age, the food they eat without having given it a thought before now seems to go from the lips to the hips, or the belly. No matter what we try to do it just leads to a steady increase in our body weight and size. It is like you have become a whole new being and you can't seem to make sense of the new you.

The unfortunate truth is that for many in the western world, that age has become earlier and earlier to the point that for some, it is now the teenage years. It seems to have become an uncontrollable problem that leads to poor self-worth and depression, which is temporarily eased by eating more to make you feel better.

It seems to me that we have been set up for failure in this area. If you are one of the fortunate people who have a fast metabolism and you can eat what you like, we say to you, God bless you. You are truly blessed as you don't have to struggle with the curse of bad genes that the majority of the population has to deal with.

So what I am trying to say is, yes, the struggle is real and IT'S HARD. There is no easy way around this problem. But what do you do? You can give up and say it is all too hard, and watch the pounds accumulate and steal your life before your eyes or you can fight to save your sanity, your body, and yes, your life.

Yes, It Is Hard, but it is not an unwinnable war.
I would like to take a moment to talk about why it is hard, in my opinion.

The way I see it, we have a number of issues that have lined up to make losing those unwelcome pounds/kilos so difficult.

1. Lifestyle and Culture
2. The Commercial Conspiracy
3. The Carb Problem
4. You

Lifestyle and Culture

Lifestyle and Culture are pervasive and the truth is that you and I are part of the problem. The western world has accepted a low activity lifestyle and high energy diet and it is generally accepted in normal land that this is just how it is.

It has become a cultural issue, and I liken cultural issues to a fish in a fish tank. Does a fish know that he is wet? To the fish, he is immersed in his environment and the only way he is aware of the fact that he is wet is when he is lifted out of his environment and he gets a different perspective.

I hope that through this book, I will attempt to take your mind on a journey and give you a different perspective that may empower you to make some choices that can change your life for the better.

Not that I have conquered this problem fully myself. I have a daily struggle to make the good decisions for my life. Sometimes I win, sometimes I lose, but in balance I am winning the battle.

The Commercial Conspiracy

Well it probably isn't a conspiracy in the traditional sense, but when you think about it, it is natural and it is conspired, unintentionally to make eating well a difficult task.

Fast food chains and food sellers generally are in the business of making money out of selling food to customers like you and I who have time constraints. Being astute business people, they work to bring customers back time and time again by providing a service and experience that is repeatable, enjoyable and profitable.

Naturally, their business model provides for foods that are inspiring to the palate, quick to devour and satisfying to the customer. Naturally they will give customers what they want, and in that demand you find bread (often sweetened), potato chips, sodas (soft drinks), and many other, tasty morsels that are high in energy which our bodies quickly transform to fat storage in our bodies.

You can't blame these companies because they have refined their business model and menu to give people what they want. This is not to say that we shouldn't as a society challenge the social conscience of these companies regarding their part in the fat epidemic.

But it is inevitable that if you consume these menus day after day then you will put on weight and fat.

Later in the book I will talk about strategies on how to take what's on offer and tailor it to work with you to control your weight.

The Carb Problem

I dare you to go to a grocery store, walk down the aisles and see how many foods you can buy without significant amounts of carbohydrates in them. Let's not forget the sugary drinks that are in abundance in stores and almost every eating facility that you find.

Our food manufacturing industries have found ways to put carbs into just about every food you buy. Some are there legitimately but many are there to create bulk or make the other more expensive ingredients stretch further.

That is why it is recommended that we avoid a lot of processed foods.

While our body needs a small amount of carbohydrates to function, the modern diet is overloaded with carbohydrates, and these carbohydrates are what the body turns to fat.

So in what form do we find these carbs?

So many foods are cooked in bread crumbs. Flour and sugars are added to many mass produced foods, potato and rice are in most TV dinners, and almost all snack foods have a combination of these. Pasta, confectionery, snack foods, cookies, and most drinks are all loaded with sugars.

I can hear it now, you are saying to yourself, is there anything left to eat? Absolutely there is. I am not saying that you can't have these in a controlled measure, but as you can see it is no wonder that we put weight on if we can't escape the high energy foods that are presented to us on a daily basis.

Knowledge is power though, and if you can gain the knowledge then you can make good choices. If you don't have the knowledge, you can't make the good choices that will empower you to win in this battle.

I will be sharing some of the strategies that I have used to beat the odds stacked against me.

You!!! Me!!!

Okay, now we have to get serious, it's time to meet the biggest enemy in this battle. You only have to look in a mirror to get a glimpse at the raging beast that lurks to steal your success away. I put it that way because of all the battles I have had in losing weight, the real truth is that I am my own worst enemy.

Everything that I hope to achieve hinges on me. It is imperative then that I acknowledge, accept and address this.

The truth is that you and I are gifted with

incredible power. We have the power to learn, we have the power to see things as they can be, not as they are now. And we have the power to choose. The power to choose what we do, what we eat, when we eat, the power to say YES, and the power to say NO.

We live in a society that wants us to shift the blame for things that are wrong in our life off to others, and we have lost the art of taking responsibility of our life decisions. Instead, we expect others to solve our problems for us. We turn the TV on and we hear doctors and politicians arguing about how bad the obesity problem is in the country and we expect them to find a way to fix it.

Well I am going to tell you a truth here that I can't yell it loud enough.

YOU ARE RESPONSIBLE FOR YOU.

I AM RESPONSIBLE FOR ME !!!!!!!!!!!!!!!

Don't think that your doctor can fix you. He will tell you what's wrong with your health and give you a prognosis if you stay on the path you're on, but he can't fix you. Only YOU can take the steps to make the change!

Several years ago I was diagnosed with Pre-Diabetes. Type 2 Diabetes runs in my family, all my uncles and grandparents had it, so I have a predisposition to develop it.

I can just accept that it is inevitable, or I can choose to make the changes in my life that will give me a fighting chance and ward it off as long as possible. I choose to make the changes. That is not a flippant choice, it is a quality choice that is going to cost me. I choose this not because it is easy, but because it is hard and only I can make the changes that will benefit me.

Sadly, Type 2 Diabetes is raging in our community in epidemic numbers and for that reason alone, what I share in this book is of, I believe such great value.

2 Why Do I Get Fat?

I would like you to imagine this scenario. You go to a car dealership and you want to buy a new car. They advertise the fuel consumption of the car at some amazing figure and it woos you into purchasing the car and you take it home.

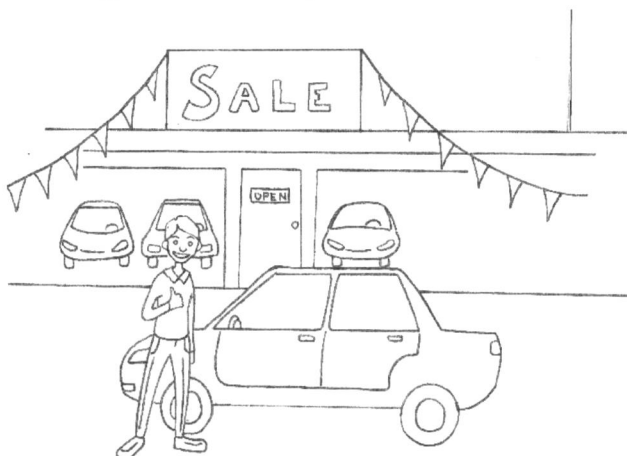

Then excitedly you want to go for a drive and

you fuel the car up and off you go. Expecting to get the advertised fuel economy of 400 miles per tank of gas, you find yourself frustrated that the car only goes 350 miles. You roll your eyes and think to yourself, "Oh well, duped again". So you carry on with your vehicle for the next couple of months, but you start to notice the car is a little bit sluggish and wallowing, and you discover that the car is actually heavier than it was when you purchased it.

You then discover, to your astonishment and annoyance, that the car seems to have these bulges under the fenders and mudguards, and padding in the doors that you were sure weren't there before. Even the trunk is looking a little bulgy.

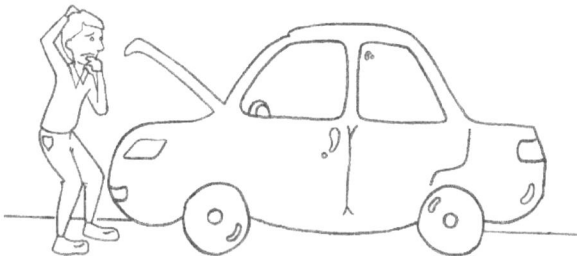

You pull out the owner's manual and start reading, and you find that there is a special feature about this car that nobody told you about.

This car takes some of the fuel from the tank every time you fill up and stores it under the car's skin for later, just in case you get stuck and can't find a fuel station.

So with this new understanding of your car's operating instructions, you start to take your car for a drive and you let the car get to empty. Lo and behold, the car keeps going for hundreds of miles and you don't need to fuel up for quite a while.

In fact, this car is quite amazing, it is designed to cover the days that you can't get to the gas station and you can just keep driving you don't even need to stop when the gauge is on empty.

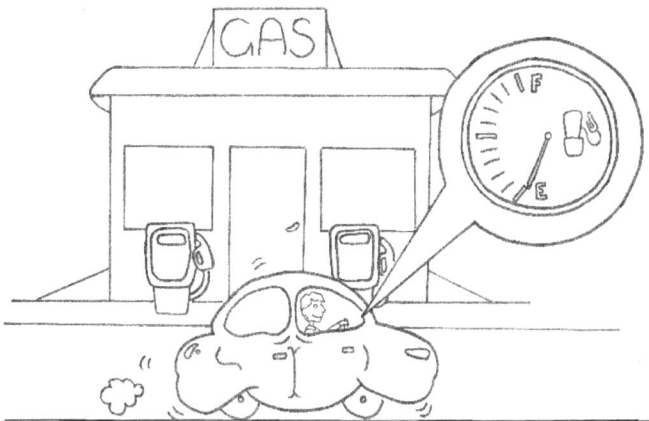

I know this little illustration is simplistic and

curious, but this is just what happens to this incredible human vehicle we have. It was created with an energy conservation system built in, so you could ride out the tough times of not being able to get food for a period of days or even up to a month.

I have to say I am in awe of this, and yet this very system is getting us into so much trouble in our current culture.

Our ancestors had to work hard to put food on the table and there would be times of leanness and times of bounty, and so this system worked wonderfully.

But fast forward to our western culture of today, food is everywhere, and if we don't get our three square meals a day we think we are hard done by. There is food everywhere that we can get in minutes, just stand in the queue and order and there it is in a couple of minutes.

Not only is our food so readily accessible, but culturally, post-modern thinking says if it feels good, do it. Foods that our bodies crave have a pleasurable side to them and so we tend not to deny ourselves that which gives us pleasure.

Add to that the fact that when our fuel gauge gets to the point that the fuel warning light comes on, it is like a huge siren going off in our heads. It grabs our very being, and tells us we have to eat or we will die, or that is what it feels like to us.

Again, we hear the familiar strains of "It's not my fault, I blame Anybody but me". I know I'm harping on this point, but our culture has been allowed to develop a Me above all things or a victim mentality.

The truth is we are talking about our health and this is a far too important part of our lives to be playing the blame game.

There are no shortages of players to blame, from fast food companies, to grocery stores, farmers to health councils, doctors and schools, but inevitably only one person is responsible for what you put into your mouth and one person who can do something about it.

To not do something about it is to give up and allow your body to become the victim of neglect.

It also has the possibility of paying you back, with all sorts of ailments. From heart disease, stroke, arthritis, type 2 diabetes, amputations, not to mention, depression, being unable to be active, lack of sex drive and poor self-esteem.

How many of you right now, reading this can identify with some of these health and personal challenges.

So what hope do we have with all this stacked against us?

Well, I am the ultimate optimist. I actually believe that human beings, ordinary men and women are actually created extraordinary. I actually believe that you are capable of great things. I believe that, like pioneers of old, there is something better just around the corner, but I know I will probably have to fight for it, figuratively speaking.

I also happen to believe that You are special. You are created and are special, so special that the challenge, should you choose to accept it, is not only Mission Possible, but undoubtedly achievable.

3 Take Ownership

With that in mind I encourage you to do what I had to do. Take ownership and responsibility for the circumstance you are in now.

If you are a few pounds overweight, or fully obese, acknowledge the fact that you are and place a stake in the ground and say:

"Enough is Enough! Today, I will take action and responsibility, and I will make the hard decisions, the tough choices that it will take to change what I have accepted up until now as fate. Now I will Take my destiny into my own hands and change my direction, from victim to overcomer, from out of control to managing my world and my diet"

"I will read on, I will learn from all sources available to me, about myself and my environment and I will take charge of my destiny"

I had to do this. If I had just let life push me around, I would have been 290lbs/130 kg by now.

I will tell you a little more about my story. I was married in 1986 at the age of 26, to the most beautiful girl in the world. At that time I was 143lb/65kg. We were two string beans and thanks to good genes, I stayed that way, able to eat anything and everything I desired and nothing seemed to change much.

Admittedly, in the first 3 months of marriage my weight went to 165lbs/75 kg, then came back down to 154lbs/70kg but it then stayed there until my mid 30's.

Then, something started to happen. First I saw a slowly developing bulge on my normally flat abs, then I noticed a slow but steady increase in my weight. Now, being a carpet cleaner, I was always on the road, eating fast food, take-away meals, drinking lots of Coke.

I didn't take much notice when I passed

165lbs/75kgs, but when I hit 176lbs/80 kg I realized that I was no longer in control of my weight. I didn't know what to do about it so I just accepted, as culturally we have been taught to do, that middle age spread is inevitable and they say it's good to have a bit of reserve on in case you need it.

I believe these are unintentional cultural white lies we tell ourselves and others to allow us to keep indulging the lifestyle we enjoy and don't want to take responsibility for. (just my opinion)

I had lost control of my weight. At my 15th wedding anniversary in June 2001, I had hit 213lbs/97kgs and I was desperate.

I thank God every day that someone put in my hand, a copy of "The New Diet Revolution" by Dr Atkins.

My wife and I read it together and took action, and by controlling the carbohydrates in my diet over the next 3-4 months, I came back to 167lbs/76kgs. I learnt so much about myself during this time and I found that what Dr Atkins had to say made so much common sense to me.

Unfortunately, there were two things he

didn't tell me, or maybe I just didn't hear what he was saying. At that point of success, thinking I had won, I let my guard down. I started reverting back to some old eating habits, not as bad as before, and slowly but surely my weight started to creep back up.

The two things were:

1. My body had now changed and it would convert any left-over energy from my food to fat very efficiently.

2. I had to continue to manage my diet even after losing the excess weight.

So these lessons are a part of what I am going to share with you in the coming pages.

Over the past 15 years I have managed my weight between 176lbs/80kgs and 198lbs/90kgs, and during that time I have learned so much about myself that I have become an expert on my own body and eating habits.

I literally have learned to steer my weight. This is a valuable lesson and I want to share that with you shortly.

So confident am I in this, that leading up to writing this book I have purposely allowed my weight to drift up to 208lbs/94.5Kg and will implement this method and blog my journey. This will show that it can be done without too much fuss, using a key tool and a bit of self-discipline.

I have shared this with you, not to boast, but hopefully to inspire you to believe that it can be done.

IF I CAN DO THIS
I AM CONVINCED THAT YOU CAN TOO

4 A Lesson From Japan

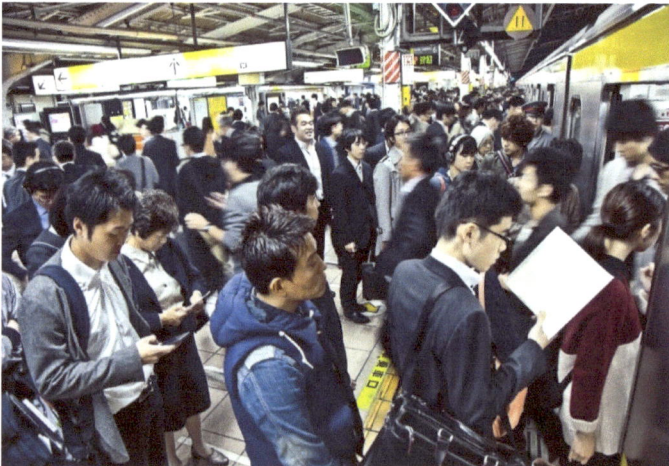

In 2015 my wife and I had the pleasure of travelling to Japan. Our son was living over there and so we spent two weeks with him in Minami

Urawa, just north of Tokyo City. During that stay we learned to ride the trains and learned a lot about the Japanese people and culture in the process.

It was an amazing eye opener for me. I saw in that environment that virtually all the people are thin, and you really have to look hard to find an overweight person. This translates into some amazing health statistics. Did you know that Japan has over 60,000 people over the age of 100? That is an astounding statistic. Not only are they over 100 but many of them are quite active in their lifestyle.

Clearly the Japanese are on to something. There are obviously many differences between Japanese culture and Western culture but I believe we can nail it down to a few key differences.

So what is it that the Japanese people do differently to us in the West?

1. They have small meal portions
2. They walk everywhere.

You can argue that this is too simple a view, but these to me are the two most glaring differences between the US, Australia, Europe and Japan.

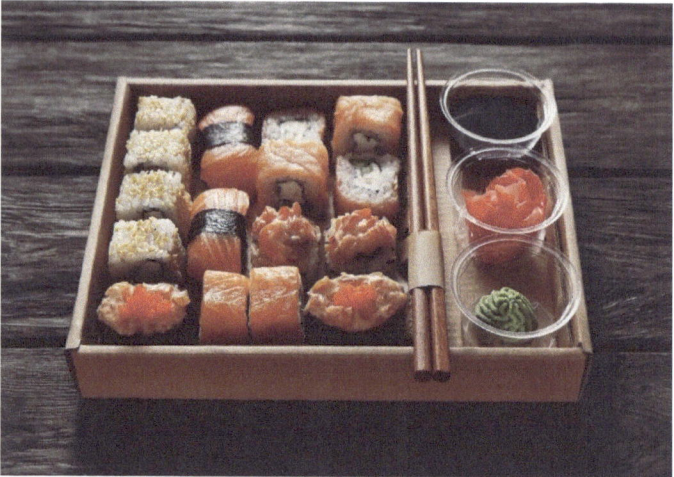

It is simple - Control Your Diet and Do Some Exercise.

We think we have been hard done by if we don't get a super-sized meal and we often eat until we are overfull. Many of us, instead of walking, get in the car at every available opportunity.

There is an advantage to living in a big city as many of you have to walk to public transport, similar to the lifestyle of the Japanese.

Taking this lesson from real life, I believe we can put into place a plan that is similar, but in our western style of doing things.

5 Make A Plan

I am a big believer in visual pictures that convey an idea,
So I want to show you how I think when it comes to what we should eat.

There are many different diets that claim to be the healthiest diet and if they work for you then I say go ahead because it's not really about being right, it is about what works for you. I have developed an illustration that works for me and guides my decision making when it comes to what I choose to eat on a daily basis.

Since discovering the Atkins style of diet I have found that I am in control of my diet to the point that like driving a car, I can steer my weight. So here is the first image I would like you to consider.

You are in control of your eating life. You sit in the driver's seat. It's your Car (Your Body) and your responsibility to negotiate the road ahead.

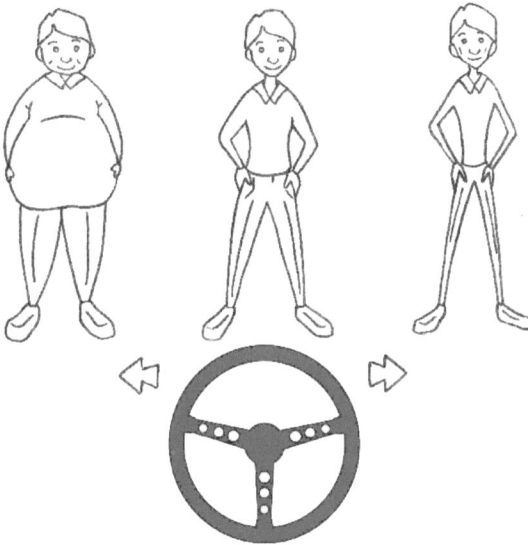

So if I steer to the right (the good foods) My weight goes down.

If I steer to the left, (the bad foods), my weight goes up.

Who is in control? YOU ARE!!

You don't hand the steering wheel over to a passenger when you are driving down the road. Nor should you when you are choosing what you eat. You take advice but ultimately it's you who drives the show.

So What Does Your Diet Look like at the Moment?

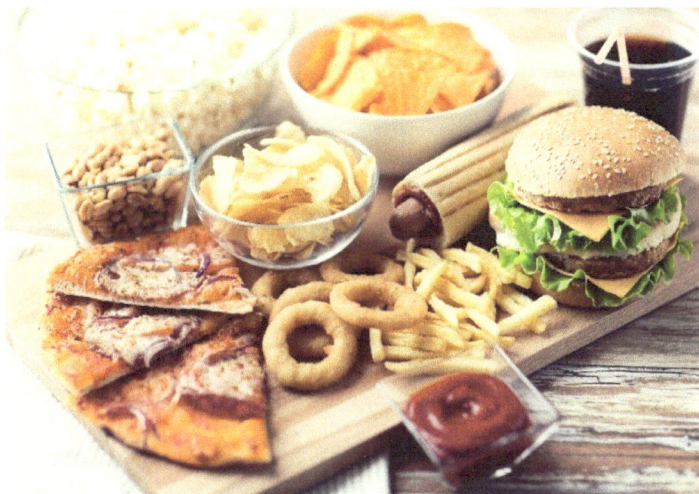

Let's stay with this illustration of driving your food life.

We know that on a two lane road you drive on your side of the center line unless you need to overtake another vehicle, right?

No one in their right mind would pull over to

the other lane to overtake then drive and stay on that side of the road for mile after mile?   You know that if you stay on that side of the road, sooner or later a car is going to come at you from the other direction and you are going to crash.

Instead, a sensible driver will drive along their side of the road and pull into the other lane for a short time only to overtake a vehicle. They will then come back to their side of the road to continue their journey safely to their destination.

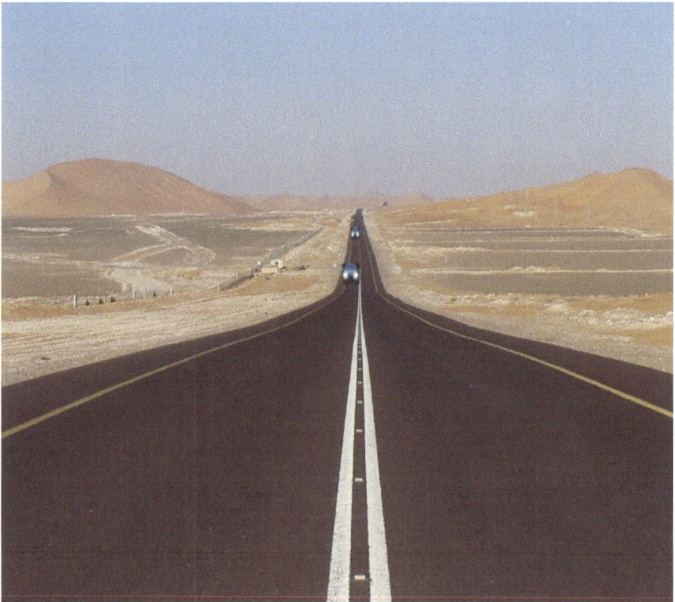

When it comes to food, we are not sensible!!!

When it comes to food, we are thrill seekers! We pull onto whichever the side of our diet road gives us the most pleasure and give No Regard to what is coming… and what is coming is not pleasant.

What is coming is the **Mobility Crash**, where we are carrying so much weight that we can't function like we should.

We also have the **Low Self Esteem Crash**, in which we look in the mirror and we just don't like what we see, and we think others are thinking the same thing. We beat ourselves up and if we let this go to its end, we end up with depression.

Then we have the Health Crashes -
High Blood Pressure,
Type 2 Diabetes,
Heart Disease, and more…

So again, who is in charge of the driving? You are!

You need to find out what you need to do to

get your life on the right side of the diet road.

Getting Down to the Plan

So, what foods do I eat regularly,
and what foods do I eat occasionally?

This is what I have found and use as a simple guide for what I choose to eat and for managing my weight.

Eat Occasionally	Eat Regularly
Most Processed Food	Most Fresh Vegetables or Natural Proteins
Sweets Confectionary	Beef
Breads	Chicken
Pasta	Pork
Sugar Based Drinks	Lamb
Cakes and Biscuits	Cheese
Rice	Eggs
Potato	Salads/Vegetables
Beer and Wines	Beans
	Avocado
Wheat Flour Products	Seafood
Fruits(See notes below)	***
Food Covered with Breadcrumbs	Foods Not Covered in Batter or Breadcrumbs

Now I can hear some of you gasping for differing reasons. Some of you can't imagine life without the left column. Some of you are saying there is so much meat in the right hand column.

Essentially the goal is to make your diet one that makes your body work for the calories rather than giving it an easy instant hit of energy which has the potential to turn easily to fat.

Your body is actually very efficient at converting the high-carb foods in the left column to usable blood sugars that give you energy. If your diet is regularly made up of a lot of these foods, your body then has to regulate these spikes of sugar by producing more of a hormone called insulin. This excess insulin is the trigger that creates fat storage in your body and consequently you put weight and bulk on.

The good news is that in regular eating of foods from the right column, the body has to use more energy to change these proteins into those usable blood sugars. Thus it is less likely to create that insulin spike which is the catalyst for the body to store fat.

I know this is simplistic and I don't claim to be an expert in this area but I can recommend a number of authors with the academic authority for you to understand this more. I just want to make it simple for you to understand my logic.

The second thing that is often raised is that the right column foods are boring. I actually couldn't disagree more. The meals available on the right column can be truly heavenly in their taste and when I am on the diet I live like a king. But remember, moderation - steer clear of having huge meals, but you can be very well fed by these dietary choices.

Her are a few examples of meals I have had lately.

Beef, Chicken or Lamb Skewers

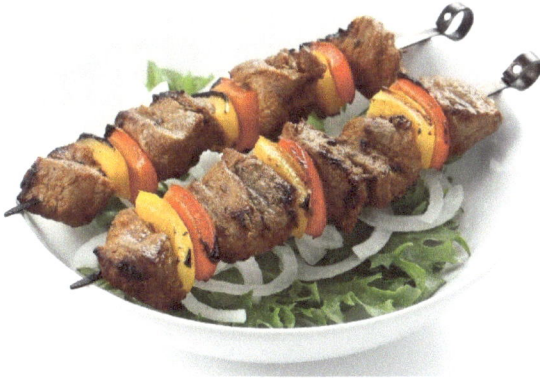

Mexican without the Tacos

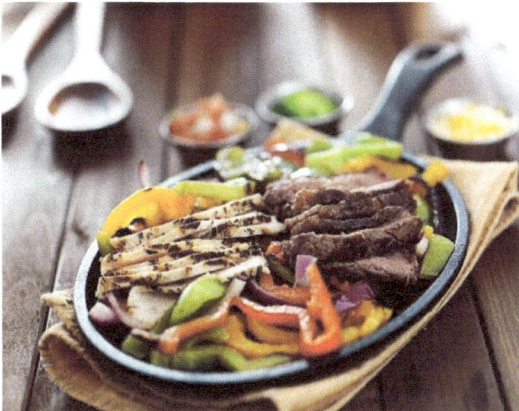

All day breakfasts

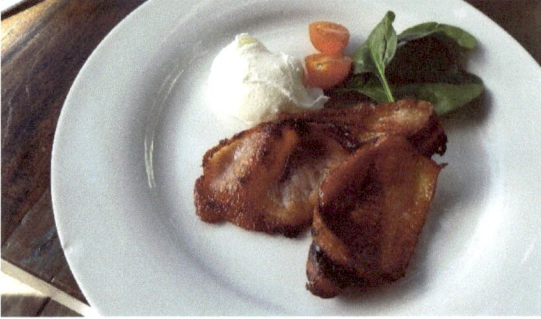

Awesome Salads

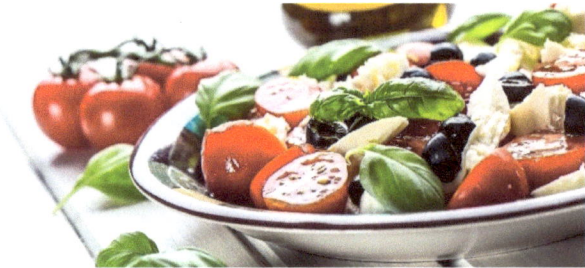

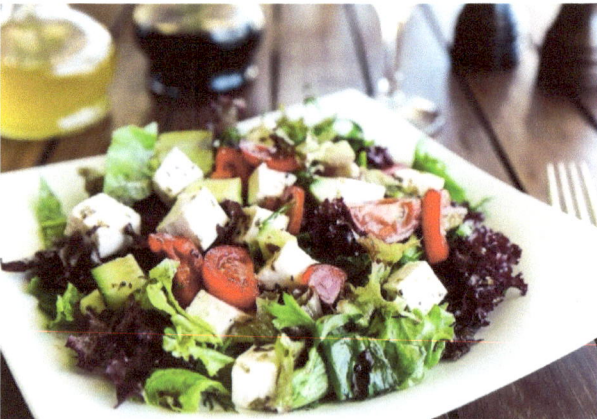

The Place of Fruits

Fruits have a special place in our diet. They have good nutritional value but so many of the fruits you eat will contain high amounts of fruit sugars, fructose, which is very easily converted into fats by the insulin spikes.

So during the weight loss period of my diet I reduce to a minimum the fruit I eat, but once I have achieved my weight goal, I introduce limited amounts of whole fruit, not fruit juice. This is because the fruit juice is high in sugars and doesn't have the natural fibers that balance out the sugars.

People who espouse the calorie restriction philosophy will actually often eat the skin and discard the center of the fruit because the nutrition is often found just below the skin and excessive calories are found in the main part of the fruit.

6 The Secret Weapon

**There is a saying in management:
"If I can measure it, I can Manage it"**

I think that of all the things I discovered when I read Dr Atkins book the Diet Revolution, the one that struck me most was that by the use of a little known device I could measure whether I was burning fat or not. To me this was a true revolution.

Every other diet I had ever looked at would say here we go, try doing ABC and eating XYZ and see how you go. There was nothing more discouraging than putting your faith in someone's recommendation only to find that you are making no long-term headway. Inevitably I would give up because the motivation was lost – I couldn't truly measure my success or properly track my progress.

So what is this amazing device that Dr Atkins recommends?

The Keto-Diastix Test Strip

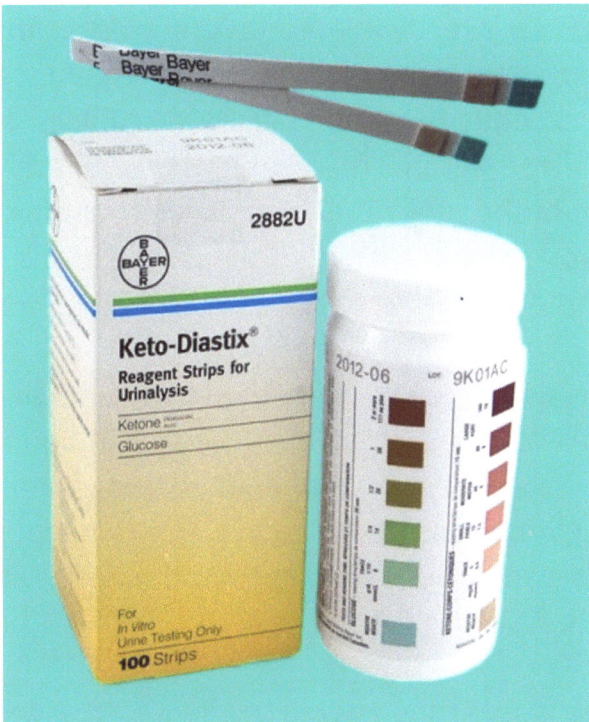

It is a KETO-DIASTIX test strip which is usually used by people with type 2 diabetes to measure if their body is functioning normally or abnormally.

A packet of 50 Keto-Diastix test strips normally retails for around $8.00, so they are not an expensive item and are available from Pharmacies, Drug Stores or even on Amazon.com.

What it is meant to do is measure the ketones in your urine. Ketones are a by-product of the chemical reaction that occurs when the body converts fats into the blood sugars that fuel our bodies. To use them just take a strip from the container and place it in the urine stream. Wait for 30 seconds to get an accurate reading of the color of the ketone reaction. If it is pale at the bottom of the range then you are not burning yet, but if you get any change to the color, from a light pink to a dark purple you are burning fat.

If you take away the source of easy sugars, e.g., lollies, cakes, chips, bread etc., the body will turn to its stored source of energy, body fat, and it will begin to consume it. When this is happening you will get a measurement on the Keto-Diastix Urine Test Strip.

The Keto Strips have a graduated color scale to show the amount of ketones detected in your urine. This will give you a guide as to the rate fat is being burned by the body at that time.

If you have been exercising heavily then you will probably have a dark purple reading on the stick, but if you have a light pink reading then you are just burning steadily.

If you are not burning any fat at all, you will have no change to the color of the keto stick.

So now we have a way to measure how effective our diet is at getting our bodies burning fat. This is an outstanding breakthrough in being able to monitor your progress on your diet.

It also gives you the ability to learn what is happening with your own body, rather than taking the advice of someone else who is just giving you their educated or uneducated opinion.

Your personal experience is the most valuable learning tool you can have in discovering exactly how your body reacts to certain foods. This can be a great moment or a distressing one depending on how much you love that food and if you get a positive or negative reading. But you can't argue with what you are finding out by this method as the Keto Strip doesn't lie.

How I Use the Keto Test Strips

One thing I might mention here, when you first get your test strips you are eager to see your test go positive for burning fat, I know I might check myself 4 times a day to make sure I am still burning, but the truth is you only need to test once a day to see if you are producing ketones as once your in the zone you will stay there if you stay on track with your diet.

Okay, so again my car images come into the game. I use the Keto-Diastix strips like a speedometer on my car. You can sit there all you like with the engine running, but if the car isn't moving forward then it won't register on the speedometer.

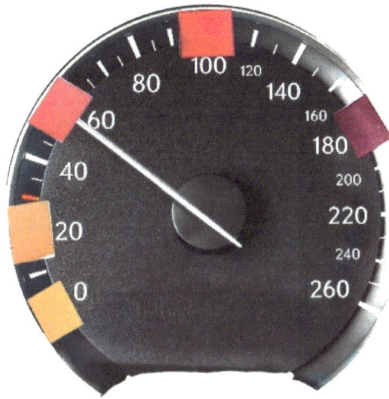

It's the same thing with the Keto strips - if you aren't burning fat, then you are going nowhere on your diet. You have to get your diet to the place that you see the colors on the keto sticks that indicate you have started burning fat. I talk about this in more detail in the next chapter.

Essentially this tool gives you the ability to measure your progress and you have something to aim for. I like to go hard at it straight away, which means decisively choosing to make this diet work, starting strong and getting the body burning solidly. Which means Dark Pink to Purple is the initial goal.

Note that every bit of exercise you do will help achieve this so try to be active in some way or another. Walking is fantastic if you can do it for

30 minutes or more a day.

Once you have achieved that positive rate of fat burning, you will start to feel so positive at having achieved even this first step. Most diets don't give you a way to know that you are burning fat. Most of them are wishy washy and lots of guess work which discourages you when you don't see the scales moving. This is a huge achievement and you will tend to stay motivated if you know the hunger and lethargy (from the sugar crash in your system) are worth it, in the end the breakthrough is worthwhile.

As long as your testing shows you have ketones in your urine then you will know that you are burning fat.

Now this is where you will begin to learn about the foods you eat. The Keto strips will let you know very quickly if the food you recently consumed had carbohydrates of any substance, because you will almost immediately stop burning fat.

Believe me, after you have been burning, to see that 'speedometer' go to zero is a real wake up call, because if you want this enough, you will soon realize that you just can't eat those foods and still lose weight.

This is a good thing because it's not some third party telling you what you can and can't eat. You are teaching yourself and I believe there is real power in that.

7 Implementation

"If it's going to BE, it's up to ME"

"Okay, this is where the rubber meets the road. Today is the most important day. It's the day that I start my diet."

Before you start, it's time to weigh yourself and measure your waist and hips. You need to be able to measure the success you are going to achieve.

"Having done all the mental preparation, I know my plan. Today I start to implement what I have planned in my mind."

The saying you use today and over the next few days is "Hunger is my friend". You know that your body is going to scream at you, "WHAT ARE YOU DOING?" And you need to very firmly put it in its place and say "I'm In Charge Here. Hunger Is My Friend."

GOAL No 1 – Fasting for 48 Hours

This first day starts like any other day, but with one exception - you decide not to eat. You are fasting for at least 24 hours, but 48 hours is good if you can do it.   The goal is to switch your body into ketosis, which you will test for using the Urine Test Strip I referred to earlier.

One thing that will happen is that the blood sugar levels your body has been used to will drop through the floor over the 48 hours. This is to be expected as you have been feeding your body unending amounts of carbohydrates that it quickly turns to energy. Now you are wanting to reset your body to draw on a more sustained form of energy from the stored fats in your body.

During this time be sure to drink water and try to avoid diet drinks during this time as you will get gassy on the inside. I like to have a cup of black tea - No Sugar - as it soothes the tummy and is refreshing.

Soon you will get that hungry sensation gnawing at you, but this is a very important sensation to resist. When I am feeling hungry, I use that saying "Hunger is my friend". I use it as a mind trick, repeating it to myself over and over again until it is like a switch gets flicked in my brain. Now I am in control. In fact, this is very important because you have to take authority over your body and not be driven by its every desire.

If you lose this battle you will lose the war.

Now in truth and honesty, if you find that you are absolutely in need of eating something, make sure it is in the protein food group. One of my favorite foods for this is chicken on a stick (called kebabs in Australia). As long as they are not covered in breadcrumbs, they are tasty, and won't feed the sugar cycle in your body that can stop you achieving your Ketosis in the 48-hour period. Another snack you can make yourself is scrambled eggs with bacon and onions, as long as you make it without adding milk to the contents. Milk has carbs that you don't need right now.

I have also found nuts to be a good food to

take away the hunger pangs, but don't eat too many as they are high in energy and they can also encourage your bowels to move.

Now a word of warning. During these 48 hours your body will be in a state of change so you may experience diarrhea, or at least a change in your bowel motions. This will settle down, and if anything, as we get into the diet, you will find that you don't have as many motions as normal and you can become constipated. That is why, when you start eating again, having salad vegetables is important to keep this part of your health in balance.

Now, Let the celebrations begin! No, I'm kidding, but be happy, because I guarantee that after these 48 hours you will now be in ketosis. You can prove it by testing your urine with the Keto test strip, which should show a pink to purple color on the test strip.

Now you are Burning Fat!
Every moment of the day that you have a reading on the Keto test strip, you are burning fat.

It's time to hop on the scales and weigh yourself. You will find that you will have dropped

1-3 kilos. This is usually a shock to you and you want to start celebrating, but sadly, this is not fat you have lost, it's just your body readjusting to the new diet. To a large degree all you have done is just lost some fluids and cleaned out your intestinal tract. But still, it is a great motivator to see the scales going in the right direction.

GOAL No 2 – Keep Yourself Burning

The goal now, is to introduce food back into your diet and to keep your body in ketosis.

Dr Michael Mosley, whom I mentioned earlier in this book, has investigated fasting and calorie restriction, and has some very good ideas in regard to this area. I have taken some of those ideas and implemented them in my daily plan.

We want to reduce the total calorie intake for the day, so I personally find it easiest to not eat until lunch time. I know this goes against the grain of what many dietitians recommend, but I have to stop putting food in my mouth. If I get into the habit of waiting till lunch time, that is a whole lot of calories that I don't consume up front.

What I do is I have a really good meal at lunch,

not too big. Using this method, I find that I really appreciate that first meal of the day and it can be very satisfying.

Once I am into fat burning mode, I find that my body doesn't get the sugar cravings that occur when eating carbs – no more spikes in blood sugar! So I don't have the craving to snack, which is very important if I am going to limit the eating.

So what sort of meals do I eat now?

My favorite meals are based around pure protein and low carb vegetables. If I am dining out, I like all day breakfasts, like:

Bacon/Sausages/Salmon and Eggs with Tomato and Mushrooms

Or

Chicken/Steak/Pork with Salads, or Caesar Salads without the Croutons. Or even Salads by themselves are extra good.

What about the FAST FOODS?

Okay, I hear you saying, what about the fast foods? Well the above rules apply when at McDonalds or KFC or any of the fast food stores.

Because many of these places have set menus, the pressure is on you to take what they offer without question, but if you know what you want, then you can order just what you want. Fast Food places are like a food factory and that includes service, If you get in line or drive thru and you haven't prepared yourself what foods you can and can't eat, the pressure of having to make an order will tend to make you choose something easy and not good for you. Don't be pressured - this is too important. Do your research and know what you want before you go up to the counter and choose your foods using the above as a guide.

My cardinal fast food rules are:

NO POTATO
NO BREAD
NO RICE
NO PASTA
NO SUGAR-BASED DRINKS

I like to be very strict on myself for about 2

weeks and by then I am in steady fat burning mode and have lost 2-4 real kilograms in weight. I will have seen the tape measure come down by an inch or so around my waist.

THIS IS WHERE THE EDUCATION BEGINS

Now, when I make the blanket statement "No Bread", it is not absolute. The reason I say this, is that now you are in the education mode of your eating. I can tell you all day what to eat and what not to eat, but if you are using your Keto Test Strips, you will learn that every bit of carbohydrate that you eat has a price and it will stop you burning fat for a period of time.

You need to understand that your body will burn carbs over any other food source. If you have a small chips with your meal, as soon as your body digests and absorbs those carbs, you will not burn fat.

But if you are wise, you will use the readings on the Keto Test Strips to guide your eating habits until you become familiar with what you can and can't get away with.

Ultimately, your goal is to burn fat, so you need to make quality decisions that will allow you to reach your goal.

Beware - Watch Out For This

When you have been on the diet for about a month to six weeks, you will start to see your weight loss slow down or stop.

This is due to the wonders of our body at work. It has recognized that the overload of carbohydrates has disappeared, and now it starts to adjust to the new balance of food that is being consumed.

It is now that you have to be on your guard because the mind games tend to begin. We can get down on ourselves because we aren't losing weight like we were, and there is an imposing feeling of wanting to give up.

Don't despair! Your body is just getting more efficient at converting the protein and vegetables to the needed energy for your body and so now you will have to re-adjust your diet a little to account for this.

When I reached this point, I found it to be a discouraging moment in the diet because nothing seems to be happening. But just stay on course and keep testing with the keto test strips and adjust your eating to ensure it stays in the fat burning side. Even if it is only the light pink color on the test strip it means you are in the zone.

Whatever you do, this is when you must not give up! Once you are through this period of a week or two, you will find a routine in the diet that just works.

It's not the choices you make when it is easy that make the difference, but the choices you make when it's tough that really count.

I actually like to settle at a loss rate of ½ lb./230g to a pound/460g a week. This may seem quite a slow rate, but remember that the weight gain that you are countering, in most cases, grew steadily over years. So it isn't a race, but a careful change to the diet to continue to see your weight steadily decline to your goal weight.

No matter what I say you will get on the scales every day no doubt to check your weight, but the real motivator is when you run the tape measure around your waist and you begin to see the inches/cm's come down.

You will start to feel better in yourself too. Partly

in a sense of achievement, but also your body feels better in its functioning as the weight drops off.

8 EXERCISE – The Next Big Secret

Now if you are like me, you get so frustrated doing something if you are getting no results. When you are eating a high carb diet, any exercise simply burns the excess carbs you have fed your body, unless you are doing some very rigorous exercise.

So, what I am about to tell you will be amazing.

When you are in Ketosis/Fat Burning mode, every bit of exercise you do will burn fat!

So,

Go for a walk –	**You will burn fat**
Mow the lawn –	**You will burn fat.**
Go to the gym –	**You will burn fat**
Play a sport –	**You will burn fat**
Ride a bike –	**You will burn fat**

DO SOMETHING – YOU WILL BURN FAT

EVEN IN YOUR SLEEP - YOU WILL BURN FAT

GET THE MESSAGE?

This is what I love about this low carb diet. You can know day in day out that you are burning fat, and if you want to accelerate it, just do something physical and see it come off faster!

SEEING SUCCESS COME YOUR WAY

Now, if you stay the course, you will be able to see and measure your success.

I like to focus my diet for about 3-4 months, but really you are wanting to change your lifestyle to have long term control of your weight.

As I write this book, I am implementing the diet to prove that it can be done. I am not just telling people what to do but leading the way by doing it. Watch my Video on FastFoodDiet.com.

During these 3 months my goal is to go from 94.5kgs down to 84kgs. That is a loss of 10kgs in 13 weeks, an average of roughly 0.75kgs per week. But my ultimate goal is to get to 74kg, which is good for my build. I know at that weight, my energy levels are higher, my blood pressure is under control and I feel good.

This goal is entirely achievable, but it is really up to you how fast or slow you achieve your weight loss goal. As long as you balance your eating to keep you just at the fat burning level, then your fat will burn and weight will come down.

9 Plan For Success

Now, if you have stayed the course and reached your goal weight – well done! But you must resist the temptation to have a celebratory feast because you will have a high chance of falling off the wagon, so to speak.

I know because it happened to me. I remember the day after losing about 22lbs/10kg, my diet was being interrupted by some family celebrations, and my brother and I went down the fuel station to fuel up his car. While I was there, I thought, "I'll just get myself a chocolate bar".

Well do you know, I almost audibly heard my brain go, "That's it, it's open slather again!". I had allowed my mind, which I had disciplined and controlled so well, to have an out. I started a chocolate binge, and before I knew it, I had put on 11lbs/5kgs.

It is so very important to have a maintenance or ongoing success plan for our mind to adjust to when we achieve our goal weight. A plan will allow the occasional indulgence, but will keep you on the right side of the road for the most part.

Remember, I said that you don't have to stay on the good side all the time, but you don't now want to stay on the bad side of the diet road. If you do, you will crash and you will fall back into old habits.

So it's important to continue to plan your eating even when you achieve your Weight Goal.

It is all about changing habits so there is less temptation to binge or go back to burgers and fries.

One of the reasons I don't tell people to do the 'Biggest Loser' thing is that if your normal life doesn't include significant exercise, then your weight control must be done with your normal life style.

Now don't get me wrong, if you love the new exercise regimen that you have developed, then absolutely go down that road. I applaud you and cheer you on.

But what about those of us that don't have a bent toward exercise? Well, we have to actively manage and be in control of our diet to make sure we don't pour too many calories into our bodies for the long haul.

Steering Your Weight and Health

So in truth, this diet and the conscious management of the diet using the Model I shared of the foods to eat regularly and the foods to eat only occasionally - this is the model for the rest of your life.

Remember, you now have the knowledge to truly be in the driver's seat - you have a license to drive your own body.

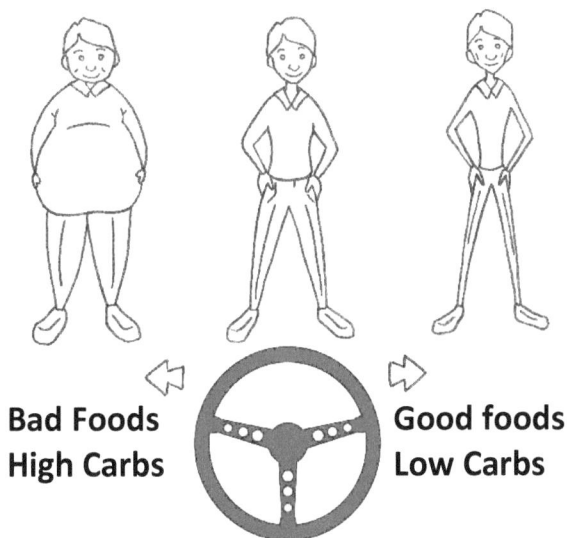

Bad Foods
High Carbs

Good foods
Low Carbs

Steer towards the high carb foods - you know your weight will go up. Steer towards the low carb foods - your weight will come down.

You are now in control. You don't have to worry about your weight any more. You have the knowledge to enjoy your life and get on with other more important things, like fulfilling dreams, enjoying friends, and living life to the full as you were created to do.

10 Summing Up

So what have we learned during this book.

1. **Be honest with yourself** about the problem that is confronting us personally and our society. Once we have a starting point and a perspective, we have a place to start our own journey

2. **Put up your hand and acknowledge that it is you/me alone who have the power to change things in our lives.** We

cannot get into the blame game. Take this quote to the bank – "If it's going to be it's up to me"

3. **Take a look at what you are going to do to change your future.** If this book has been a help to you, I hope that is has simplified the potential process and given you hope that you can do it too.

4. **Remember, You have the right and the obligation to be the Expert on You.** Learn about yourself and how your body reacts so you have control.

5. **With a simple plan of action, you can now chose the foods** you eat based on whether the food is going to take you down the low carbohydrate route and lose weight or the high carbohydrate route and allow the weight to keep piling on. Remember the crash is inevitable if you cruise on the wrong side of the diet road.

6. **With a simple way to measure our success** and monitor it on a daily basis using the Keto Test Strips to know that you know whether you are burning fat

or not and that knowledge gives you the ability to take action to keep yourself on the road to burning fat consistently. Remember, with this knowledge it enables you to become an expert on you. Learn what works for you and then take that knowledge to empower your control over your own weight management story.

7. **Plan for the future once you have reached your weight goals** so it doesn't happen again. It is critical that you don't fall back into bad habits but you manage your diet and make wise choices into the future so the monster of weight gain doesn't have its way with you again.

8. **This one is the most important of all.** If you find you have fallen off the wagon and got back into old habits. It is never too late to come back and make it happen all over again. Failure is not failure unless you quit. Make a decision not to give up but to keep at it until you succeed.

**Good Luck and God's Blessing
on you in your journey.**

Notes

I recommend these books to read if you want more detailed knowledge of low carb diets a and calorie restriction.

Dr. Atkins' New Diet Revolution
https://www.amazon.com/Dr-Atkins-New-Diet-Revolution/dp/006001203X/&tag=dietgoodideas-20

QR Code

The 8-Week Blood Sugar Diet: How to Beat Diabetes Fast (and Stay Off Medication)
Michael Mosley

https://www.amazon.com/8-Week-Blood-Sugar-Diet-medication/dp/1501111221/&tag=dietgoodideas-20

QR Code

Contact Peter MacDonald on
Facebook
https://www.facebook.com/myfastfooddiet/

QR Code

Peter MacDonald's Amazon Author Page

https://www.amazon.com/Peter-
MacDonald/e/B00EHBU0N0/&tag=dietgoodideas-20

QR Code

www.ingramcontent.com/pod-product-compliance
Lightning Source LLC
Chambersburg PA
CBHW041214270326
41930CB00001B/12

* 9 7 8 0 9 9 5 4 3 6 2 0 6 *